7-Day
Sleep Challenge

7-Day

SLEEP

CHALLENGE

Sleep Better In 7 Days

CHALLENGE SELF

http://www.ChallengeSelf.com

Challenging Publishing

ISBN 978-1-796-66425-6

Printed in the United States of America

First Edition

YOUR OVERVIEW:

Your Instructions: How to Best Approach This - 9

Your Challenge: Get Better Sleep - 13

DAY 1: Sleep Deterrent Disposal - 17
☐ *Toxic Consumption Cleanse - 17*
☐ *Sleep-Aid Foods - 21*
☐ *Healthy Meal Plan - 24*
☐ *Exercise: Filter Innutritious Junk - 26*

DAY 2: Sleep Environment Upgrade - 29
☐ *Bedroom Makeover - 29*
☐ *Temperature Balance - 31*
☐ *Better Bed for Better Sleep - 32*
☐ *Exercise: Keep Bedroom Tidy - 34*

DAY 3: Sleep Aid Hacks - 37

☐ *Delicate Dwelling - 37*

☐ *Aromatherapy Sleep-Induced Hack - 39*

☐ *Aerial Induced-Sleep Hack - 41*

☐ *Visual Sleep-Induced Hack - 43*

☐ *Exercise: Speed Up Sleep - 44*

DAY 4: Sleep Preparation Ritual - 47

☐ *Guided Sleep Plan - 47*

☐ *Sleepwear Mental Anchoring - 50*

☐ *Exercise: Initiate Sleep Mode - 52*

DAY 5: Sleep Practical Applications - 55

☐ *The Holistic Factors - 55*

☐ *Breathing Meditation - 57*

☐ *Yoga Pose 1: The Wide-Angle Seated Pose - 58*

☐ *Yoga Pose 2: The Locust Pose - 59*

☐ *Yoga Pose 3: The Child's Pose - 61*

☐ *Powerful Sleep-Induced Sounds - 62*

☐ *Exercise: Calm Down Calamity - 65*

DAY 6: Sleep Behavioral Modification - 69

☐ *Daily Structural Changes* - 69

☐ *Early Bird Conversion* - 72

☐ *Exercise: Set Each Period's Performance Level* - 75

DAY 7: Sleep Pattern Establishment - 77

☐ *Relaxation Therapy* - 77

☐ *Sleep Assessment Exercise 1: Break Habits* - 80

☐ *Sleep Assessment Exercise 2: Rest Body* - 81

☐ *Sleep Assessment Exercise 3: Follow Routine* - 82

☐ *Sleep Assessment Exercise 4: Automate Activities* - 83

☐ *Sleep Assessment Exercise 5: Relieve Muscles* - 84

☐ *Final Experimentation: Week Schedule Ahead* - 85

Challenge Complete: Awaken Refreshed - 97

Your Feedback: Was Your Challenge Accomplished? - 101

Your Instructions:

How to Best Approach This

This book is not meant to be read entirely in one sitting, but for over the span of each day.

Why? The reasons are relatively simple. We do want you to benefit from the information, which will take time to process, and we do not want to overwhelm you with all the applications of what you will learn. At the same time, we don't want to make this another breezy one-time read, and then you're off to do something else, forgetting your new knowledge without ever applying it to anything.

Now you probably will be eager and tempted to go through this all in one sitting, but we're encouraging you to take it slow. Remember that the best way to approach this is <u>one day</u> at a time. Do not move on to the next day until you have completed its previous day(s).

This approach is effective because if you truly want to improve, you need to remain grounded in the process. There is no such thing as a magic pill; there is continuous conditioned improvement. Rome wasn't built in a day. Likewise, none of the top performers, best athletes, and successful people in the world have gotten to where they are in a day. Breaking things up into separate days supports an ongoing process and builds upon each previous day's progress to bring it all home in the end.

Of course, each individual's experience will be different. You may or may not accomplish your goal after the entire trial is over. In that case, you can repeat it all again starting from Day 1 to the last day.

If you commit yourself, you will see improvement. Are you ready to proceed on to your challenges? Then let's begin!

P.S. If you ever need to contact us, you can always reach out to us at our official website:
http://www.ChallengeSelf.com

<u>Your Challenge:</u>
Get Better Sleep

After a long hard day, you can't wait to climb into bed, turn off the light, and get a good night's sleep. Unfortunately, as much as you probably love, want, and need sleep, you still may not get what the doctor ordered. When you are so exhausted but you have trouble falling asleep or staying asleep, it can drive you crazy. *But we're going to help you.*

If you have a love/hate relationship with your bed because you can't sleep—**you're not alone.**

According to the **National Institutes of Health** (www.ncbi.nlm.nih.gov/books/NBK19960), 50 to 70 million people suffer from sleep disorders in the U.S. If you are one of those sleepyheads, then it's probably no surprise that research shows that poor sleep habits or sleep quality can result in reduced productivity, concentration, mental clarity, and even a decrease in your energy level.

For some people, their lifestyle is the main cause of poor sleep. For others, medical conditions could be to blame— such as hypertension, diabetes, anxiety, and depression.

Don't despair. With some natural cures and a few tips and tricks, you can be a better sleeper. And being less tired isn't the only benefit of improving your sleep. It can also help you look and feel more energetic, have better health, and have more willpower to take on any task or challenge.

Here's a good way to think about it. Suffering from insomnia is like being stuck in a dirty, rusty, and dark environment. Then a brave hero rides up gallantly on a white horse with a magic sleep formula. *Poof!* Suddenly, the world becomes clean, shiny, and oh-so-beautiful. Yes, that sounds a bit like a fairy tale, but it illustrates the dramatic improvement you can have after every night of traveling to happy slumberland. This dream can come true if you follow our advice.

It really is possible to improve your sleep quality in just seven days. *Are you ready to give it a try?*

Now please bear in mind—our sleep methods are not intended to replace the <u>advice</u> of your doctor or other medical professionals. If you have been prescribed any medicine for a sleep disorder, please continue with the treatment. In fact, we believe that our regimen could be a great addition to your doctor's advice. Or, if you prefer, you may begin our sleep plan once your current treatment is complete.

DAY 1:

Sleep Deterrent Disposal

Toxic Consumption Cleanse

If your sleep quality is not so good—start by taking a closer look at **your lifestyle**. It is true that factors like stress, depression, and anxiety are often caused by things that are out of our control. Of course, just going to work can be stressful.

But the good news is you can decrease the effects of these factors by simply getting rid of anything "toxic" that can make you, for instance, too excited, too full, or too nervous at night.

According to Dr. Russel Rosenberg from the National Sleep Foundation, there are certain types of **foods** *you should avoid* if you want to sleep better at night. It's no surprise that you should try to avoid anything with caffeine in it. But you should also stay away from food with too much fat or sugar.

Therefore, your assignment on **Day 1** is to remove any sleep-districting foods from your kitchen or anywhere else that you may store food, so you are not tempted. Be sure to check everywhere:

Pantry: Toxic liquids like wine and other alcoholic beverages, coffee, and other caffeinated drinks, as well as toxic snacks including anything you may eat too close to bedtime or that could have an effect on your sleep need to go. Do you love having a cup of joe after dinner? *Stop!* How about some dark chocolate for dessert? *Stop!*

Dispose of those caffeinated drinks and snacks now. They are known to be stimulants, which can hamper your sleep or make you wake up several times throughout the night.

Refrigerator: Do the same thing in your refrigerator. Toss out any toxic beverages (soda, beer, *etc.*) or toxic snacks that you might be tempted to consume at night. What about one more slice of pie or another cookie before going to bed? *Just don't do it!* Dr. Rosenberg says when you eat fried or fatty food before bed, it can cause acid reflux which keeps you awake.

Freezer: Now open up your freezer and ditch any frozen foods that are high in sugar, fat, or caffeine.

Now that you've tossed out the offending food and drinks, follow these recommendations:

- Make sure you don't eat any of the toxic foods on Day 1. Instead of the bad snacks, choose healthier options such as fruits and veggies. Be sure to stay away from fast food.

- For drinks, it's best to stick with water today. If you love coffee, it's okay to have <u>one cup</u> today as long as it's <u>early in the morning</u>. Remember, if you drink coffee or anything else with caffeine in it in the afternoon or evening, you'll increase your risk of a sleepless night.

The things that you do to modify your eating and drinking on Day 1 may seem difficult at first if you're used to eating junk food and chugging lots of soda and coffee throughout the day. But once you come to realize how much better you will sleep, these changes can easily become part of your daily routine.

When you want to improve your sleep habits, modifying your eating is always a good first step because food (especially unhealthy food) can have such a long-lasting impact on your body when it comes to your weight, digestion, and discomfort after meals.

Sleep–Aid Foods

Now that we've told you what types of food you *can't* eat, let's focus on some of the great things you *can* eat.

Here's a list of foods you can look forward to eating for meals or snacks:

Cherries: Registered dietitian and nutritionist Keri Gans in New York recommends drinking tart cherry juice at night because it can help improve your sleep duration. Cherries contain melatonin—a hormone that triggers sleepiness during night hours.

Milk: Did your parents or grandparents ever recommend drinking a cup of warm milk before bed? You should have listened to them! Milk contains an amino acid called "tryptophan," which is a precursor to a chemical found in the brain called "serotonin," which helps regulate sleep.

Jasmine rice: Not only is jasmine rice delicious, but it also has been proven to be beneficial for sleep. That's because it is digested slowly by the body, so the glucose contained in the rice is released gradually into the bloodstream. So, instead of feeling hyper and uneasy after a good meal, you'll feel more tempted to go to sleep.

Fortified cereal: Carbohydrates are said to be good for sleep. If you consume one big bowl of cereal a few hours before sleep, you will improve your chance of sleeping like a baby. Of course, you're better off picking a healthy cereal, not one that's loaded with sugar.

Bananas: Bananas taste great and help promote sleep because they're rich in magnesium and potassium, which are natural muscle relaxants.

Turkey: After a huge meal on Thanksgiving, don't you feel like plopping down on the couch and falling asleep? That's because turkey is rich in *tryptophan*, just like we said with milk.

***Valerian tea**: This is a great alternative to drinking coffee at night. Valerian tea is known to have some mild sedative characteristics found in valerian acids. Also, note that this tea is known to help fight insomnia.

***Chamomile tea**: Here's another great tea option. Chamomile tea is known to have powerful anti-inflammatory and antispasmodic properties. Enjoy a cup 30 minutes before bed.

*<u>Note</u>: Regarding drinking tea before bed, don't drink too much or else your sleep will be disrupted by the frequent trip to the toilet. Drink only a small amount with the tea as potent as possible is recommended.

Healthy Meal Plan

Now that you have a list of foods and drinks that will help you sleep better, you need a plan for how to introduce them into your life. *It's easy.*

For foods that are big enough to count as a meal—or can easily be combined with others to make a meal—you should eat them more frequently.

If it's dinner, try to eat at least three hours *before* bedtime because you don't want to try to sleep right when your stomach is starting to digest all that food. For snacks or drinks, you can have those 30 minutes to one hour *before* sleep for the best effects. You can eat those closer to bedtime because they are lighter and can be digested quickly.

So, for **liquids** such as <u>valerian/chamomile tea, milk, and cherry juice</u>:

- Drink them at night, all week, a few minutes before going to bed. For variety, you can opt for tea three days a week, warm milk two days a week, and cherry juice two days a week—depending on your specific preferences.

For **light snacks** like <u>bananas and fortified cereals</u>:

- Eat them twice a week, on alternating days, before bed.

For **heavier foods** like <u>jasmine rice and turkey</u>:

- Save them for the middle of the week when you could be stressed out and anxious for whatever reason. This will help remind you that a good night's sleep can help you carry on. So, days like Tuesday, Wednesday, and Thursday could be your days for turkey, rice, or similar foods.

This variety of sleep-friendly foods and beverages spread out throughout the week will fill you up, help you relax, and make it easier for you to fall asleep and stay asleep.

Exercise: Filter Innutritious Junk

Let's review Day 1 so you can put this plan into action.

First, get rid of all those toxic foods. Be sure to check your pantry, refrigerator, freezer, and even the secret snack drawer in your desk! Dump anything containing too much fat, sugar, caffeine, or alcohol.

Next, set up your plan of how you will add the good foods and drinks to your weekly routine. Remember all the items we've suggested, such as turkey, jasmine rice, chamomile tea, and warm milk.

Don't forget that you should not eat *any* of the toxic foods on day one.

DAY 2:

Sleep Environment Upgrade

Bedroom Makeover

Time for **Day 2**—this is the day you will give your bedroom a *makeover*.

If you have a lot of unnecessary things in your room, then you already don't have an optimum environment for sleeping. *Why is that?* You need fresh and clean air to breathe, especially while you're sleeping.

Some people opt for sleeping with their window slightly open for ventilation, which is fine as long as you don't live in a heavily polluted city. However, decluttering your bedroom will give you better results to minimize the risk of inhaling mold, dust, or any bad odors in your room.

There are essentially three things you need to do when decluttering your bedroom, and they are organizing, disposing, and recycling.

- **Organizing.** Box up anything in your bedroom that's unnecessary and store those boxes somewhere else, such as in the garage, basement, or attic.

- **Disposing.** Throw away anything in your bedroom that you don't need anymore (any trash such as empty cans or food containers). Don't just throw them in a trash can in your bedroom. Get the trash out of your house.

- **Recycling.** This helps create more space in your room and allows more air to come into your room. For example, if you have any boxes or plastic containers that are just taking up space, use them to store things like shoes or office supplies.

Temperature Balance

The temperature of your bedroom is another important factor. In fact, the temperature plays a huge role in the quality of your sleep. And we'll tell you why:

Just imagine that you've had trouble sleeping for the past couple of months, and then suddenly one night you manage to fall into a deep sleep. Two hours later, you wake up because it's either too hot or too cold. So you decide to hop out of bed and adjust the temperature. That's okay, but when you climb back into bed, it's highly unlikely that you'll reenter that deep sleep that was interrupted by the temperature. From there, instead of heading back into dreamland, you find yourself counting sheep, playing with your phone, or watching TV until your alarm clock rudely tells you it's time to get ready for work, only to continuously make friends with the "snooze" button.

What a tragedy!

Do yourself a favor and make sure the temperature in your room is just about right before you hit the sheets. Another way to look at it is to think of the room temperature like a stock value that will either increase or decrease as the night goes on, and you'll want to select the best moderately-balanced level so the volatility is not too huge.

Better Bed for Better Sleep

You should also have the proper bedding, mattress, and pillow. And pay attention to how you position your bed in your room. Yes, where you place your bed in the room really can make a difference!

The best place for your bed is right in the <u>center of the room</u> so it's not too close to the door or any windows. *Why the center of the room?* The main reason is to shield you from any noise or light as much as possible, plus to get more open air around the room than if you were to place it in a dark corner that lessens the amount of air being circulated. Your bed should be a restricted zone for comfort and sleep.

You can also improve your sleep by selecting the best bedding for the right sleeping conditions. *Don't worry.* We won't push you into spending a fortune on one of those really expensive orthopedic mattresses which can cost up to $1,000. There are other ways to upgrade your current bed without draining your bank account. Get yourself a **foam mattress topper** or **mattress pad**. They only cost around $15 to $25 at big discount retail stores like Target or Walmart. There are different kinds, including gel-infused (that keeps you cooler), and they're a great alternative to buying a costly new mattress.

If you are not satisfied with your pillow then get a **contour memory foam pillow**. It will adjust to the shape of your neck, head, and upper back and remain firm (which promotes keeping a straight neck while you are sleeping). Like the mattress pads, memory foam pillows are available at places like Target or Walmart for around $25.

Exercise: Keep Bedroom Tidy

After you are finished decluttering your room, your exercise for today is to learn to naturally improve bedroom ventilation for better sleeping quality at night by doing the following:

1. In the morning when you wake up, open your window and let the air get in while you are getting ready for work.

2. When you're about to leave the house, shut the window and leave your bedroom door open so the air can circulate from room to room while you're at work.

3. Finally, every night before going to sleep, make sure you've left nothing out of place in your bedroom like trash or dirty clothes on the floor, *etc.* If you keep up with this habit, you won't have to worry about clutter ever again.

DAY 3:

Sleep Aid Hacks

Delicate Dwelling

We may be so busy throughout the day that most of the time we *neglect* our sleeping space.

One thing that you should be aware of is that your bedroom is like a sanctuary. Not only is it supposed to be the safest place in the world for you, but it is also where you should be able to rest and rejuvenate your body like a power outlet for recharging your batteries.

That's why specialists like Dr. Robin S. Haight, a Virginia-based clinical psychologist, stress the importance of preparing the room where you sleep (or try to sleep) every night.

Getting your room ready means making sure that:

- Again from Day 2, the room has been aired well enough and has the right temperature *(not too cold, not too hot)*; and the bed is placed in the right position.

- Second, you do the right things before bed, such as having a cup of tea *(caffeine-free!)* or warm milk (like we recommended in Day 1), or simply taking a warm bath.

- Third, your room has an inviting and calming vibe or scent when you finally enter it at bedtime—which we will get more into next.

Aromatherapy Sleep–Induced Hack

Lying in bed for hours and not being able to sleep really stinks, *doesn't it?* But that isn't necessarily just an expression.

Literally, sometimes the smell of a room can impact your sleep. Think about it. Whether you are inside or outside, a pleasant smell can make you feel comfortable or happy, or remind you of a happy place or idea.

So why not make sure your bedroom smells good so you can sleep better?

One way to do that is to make sure that *you* smell good when you go to bed. Take a bath with natural oils in the water, or rub some oil on your wrists before going to bed. Or you can buy air fresheners which come in a variety of options including plug-ins, scent packets, and sprays.

The **recommended scents** for sleeping are very soft and inviting, such as the following:

–lavender

–chamomile

–bergamot

–jasmine

–rose

In fact, some experts have even suggested that scents like jasmine are almost *as good* as the prescription drug **Valium** for relieving anxiety and promoting sleep. (You can read up more about it here: www.sciencedaily.com/releases/2010/07/100708104320.htm.)

As an <u>alternative method</u> if you don't want to take a bath with oil or rub it on your wrist, you can make a **pillow mist** with chamomile (or one of the other oils we mentioned):

1. Combine 1/2 cup of water with 1/2 teaspoon of witch hazel and five drops of chamomile.

2. Mix/Shake in a spray bottle for 20 seconds.

3. Spray the mixture a few times on your pillow before bed.

Overall, regardless of how you decide to use aromatherapy—these scents can help you relax and let yourself go at bedtime.

Aerial Induced-Sleep Hack

There are many options for naturally enhancing your sleeping mood with scents and colors. And having the right plant in your bedroom can make a big difference.

According to Dr. Bryan Raudenbush, a psychologist from Wheeling Jesuit University in West Virginia, having certain plants in your bedroom can help you achieve greater sleep efficiency.

Here's a list of some well-known plants for sleep aid:

The spider plant: *No, there are no spiders in it!* The spider plant is recommended because of its ability to relieve headaches. You know how stress and anxiety can lead to headaches by the end of the day, and falling asleep with a splitting headache is nearly impossible.

The snake plant: *What? First a spider plant, and now a snake plant?* The snake plant is a part of NASA's clean air study and is well-known for its ability to remove common chemicals and toxins from the air, helping you to relax at night.

Aloe vera: *And you thought aloe vera was only something you would find in juice beverages and skin care products?* This perennial is known to be effective at removing benzene and formaldehyde from the air, which are respiratory irritants that could cause chest pain, shortness of breath, coughing, and nose and throat irritation (which you know can easily ruin your night's sleep).

Visual Sleep-Induced Hack

Having gone over olfactory and aerial methods to enhance your sleep, we will now give you some quick visual methods.

This should come as no surprise—**light** is one of the biggest obstacles for sleeping.

A great thing to do, especially for those who have a hard time sleeping at night, would be to turn off your phone *(don't check your email, Facebook, or Twitter while in bed!)*. Being exposed to the blue light technology emitting from your phone or electronic devices suppresses your level of the sleep-inducing hormone "melatonin," thus making it more difficult to sleep. (For those relying on your phone as a morning alarm—get a good old alarm clock.)

One more tip is to use more "sleep-inviting nightlight bulbs" in your bedroom. Consider getting dark blue, dark green, or purple bulbs. Yet, you may be surprised to hear that **"red"** is the best light for sleeping according to sleep psychologist Michael Breus, Ph.D., as well as multiple clinical studies out there involving red light therapy because it allows the body to produce more melatonin.

Try this: Concentrate on staring at a flaming red candle in the dark—then notice how sleepy you get.

Exercise: Speed Up Sleep

Here's your easy exercise for Day 3:

- Turn off the lights (or put on your night light).

- Set the right scent/vibe in your room by rubbing your oil of choice on your wrists or spraying pillow mist with your chosen scent.

- Breathe slowly counting to 20, and then count backward from 20 to one.

Goodnight!

DAY 4:

Sleep Preparation Ritual

Guided Sleep Plan

When you've decided to call it a day and hit the hay, do you give much thought to *what you wear?*

This is definitely a factor if you want to get a better night's sleep. Everything that you do before going to bed should help convince your brain that you are conditioning yourself to sleep. And that includes your choice of sleepwear because it's part of your direct sleeping environment.

In other words, this is almost like a continuation of our guidelines from the previous Day 3.

Consider how it works with children. Typically, they have a daily routine with activities and items (like clothing, books, *etc.*) that are supposed to signify something to the child. For example, eating breakfast, brushing teeth, and getting dressed is the routine before leaving for school. Usually, there's a bedtime routine too, such as taking a bath, brushing teeth, putting on pajamas, and reading a book before turning out the light.

It turns out that when you set up a routine with children, at some point in time, they will be so well-conditioned, that you won't have to tell them what to do. One day, the child may remind the parent, *"Hey! Mom/Dad, maybe it's time for me to take a bath and get ready for bed."* Do you see what we mean here?

From now on, in order to start conditioning yourself for bedtime, you should:

- Buy the proper nightwear, like pajamas, nightgowns, slippers, *etc.*, which should signal to your brain that, *"Okay, I'm tired, and I think I should get myself to sleep now."*

- Leave your sleepwear in a cozy place in your room, preferably on a chair, folded up, and in plain sight.

- Use the sleepwear that is strategically located in your bedroom as an indicator that perhaps it's time to take a bath, drink your cup of sleep-aid tea or milk, spray your pillow mist for the night, and all the other things we talked about earlier.

Once you get into this routine, seeing those pajamas on the chair in your room will cue your brain into following the steps you should take to prepare for dreamland.

Sleepwear Mental Anchoring

We can't wrap up Day 4 without showing you a few tricks on how to turn your sleepwear into "sleep-right-away tools."

This is what you should do:

1. Pick <u>five different types</u> of sleepwear that will fit with the occasion and your mood (whether you feel like wearing fancy, elaborate pajamas, or something simple like shorts and a t-shirt).

2. Remember the weather—the temperature in your bedroom is important. For example, if you like it warm when you sleep, then maybe the long pajamas are the way to go.

3. Consider the proper fabric—don't put on sleepwear that's going to make you itchy all night.

4. Then, set up your combination of pajamas and slippers on a chair.

5. Next, close your eyes and imagine you are walking on clouds in this outfit.

6. This vision should be so comfortable that you should also smell the scent that you've picked as your pillow mist (lavender, chamomile, rose, bergamot, *etc.*).

Make it a mental anchor as soon as you see or think about your sleepwear, it should take you to that vision in the clouds where your eyes are closed, and where the smell of lavender invites you to sleep. In your head, it will be the signal that it is time to sleep.

Are you feeling sleepy right now?

Exercise: Initiate Sleep Mode

For practice, follow this "sleep-right-away" mental anchoring process:

1. Set up your sleepwear.

2. Close your eyes for a few seconds and imagine yourself walking in the clouds.

3. Introduce the scent you've chosen for your pillow mist.

From now on, this is what your sleepwear should be: a reminder to turn on your *sleep mode* in progress.

DAY 5:

Sleep Practical Applications

The Holistic Factors

Your seven-day sleeping regimen would not be complete without a little bit of meditation and some soothing sounds. Mixing breathing with yoga and white noise can really benefit you at some point during the week. It has to be done a few minutes *before* sleep (preferably 10 to 15 minutes).

You probably already know that stretching exercises can help you relax your muscles and relieve anxiety. And being relaxed and less anxious is exactly what you need before trying to sleep.

According to holistic health expert Amanda LoRusso, who lived and studied at the Kripalu Center for Yoga & Health in Massachusetts for two years, yoga can improve your sleep efficiency, including:

- Your total sleep time.

- How long it actually takes you to fall asleep.

- Stopping you from waking up in the middle of the night.

So Day 5 will focus around breathing and yoga poses and then on ending the day with soothing sounds (white noises).

Breathing Meditation

For your activity before bed on Day 5, we will start by showing you some breathing and yoga techniques that will help you sleep better.

You can place a pillow on the floor or do these exercises right on your bed. Here's what to do:

1. In the seated position, breathe in raising your hands up and joining them on top of your head (this opens up your lungs to let oxygen in and prepare you for the poses).

2. Next, lower both hands on your sides and exhale slowly (lower the hands slowly, try not to make any abrupt movements).

3. Continue breathing in and out nine more times, slowly, as if you were trying to chase away all the

negativity and anxiety that prevents you from relaxing and falling asleep. After the tenth breathing cycle, start with the yoga poses that we will list below.

Now we will be going over <u>three different yoga poses</u> for a better night's sleep. You don't have to do all three of them at the same time, instead pick <u>one</u> or <u>two</u> of them (according to your preference) and alternate them per week.

Combine the breathing with these yoga poses to make the exercises far more effective.

Yoga Pose 1: The Wide-Angle Seated Pose

1. While sitting on the bed, spread your legs straight apart as wide as possible like you're attempting a split and position your pillow right in front of your torso.

2. Inhale while sitting up as tall as possible.

3. Exhale, leaning forward from the hips and walking both hands in front of you until your upper body rests on the pillow.

4. Rest while taking a deep breath on the pillow for 10 rounds.

5. End this first cycle by inhaling while slowly returning to the seated position.

This exercise should last about <u>five</u> minutes, so make sure you take your time, pushing your hands forward as much as you can without forcing or hurting yourself. It's okay if you can't go completely flat on your mattress. Remember, position the pillow right under your belly for comfort.

Yoga Pose 2: The Locust Pose

1. Begin with the same exercise described in the first pose until you are on your stomach with the pillow supporting your hips and belly.

2. While gazing at the mattress, keep the back of your neck long, interlacing your fingers behind your back.

3. Exhale while extending your arms behind you. Lift your hands toward the ceiling while pressing the top of your toes into the mattress.

4. Exhale while trying to hold that position.

5. Inhale again, lifting your chest and head, while you gaze forward with the back of your neck neutral.

6. Exhale, once again holding the position while counting to 10 breathing in and out very slowly.

7. Finally, exhale and lower your back to the bed with your hands by your sides.

Again, complete this pose with calmness and tranquility. Do not force anything, and make sure you repeat this process <u>nine</u> more times before ending this session.

Yoga Pose 3: The Child's Pose

1. Sit up on the bed with your knees bent and your lower legs folded under you.

2. Roll your torso forward and bring your forehead to rest on your bed.

3. Next, lower your chest as close to your knees as you comfortably can and extend your arms in front of you.

4. Hold the pose and breathe. (Try to hold the pose for about <u>five</u> minutes, again by breathing slowly.)

Powerful Sleep-Induced Sounds

The last thing to do for your sleep preparation for Day 5 is to use white noise also known as **"binaural beats."** Binaural beats are considered by experts like Kelly Howell—a prominent brainwave researcher known as "The Brain Whisperer"—as scientifically proven ways to speed up the sleeping process in people who suffer from insomnia.

There are basically <u>four types</u> of binaural waves or frequency patterns, as described by **Medical News Today.** (For more info about binaural beats: <u>www.medicalnewstoday.com/articles/320019.php</u>)

Delta pattern: Binaural beats in the delta pattern are set at a frequency of between <u>0.1</u> Hz and <u>4</u> Hz—which is associated with *dreamless sleep*.

Theta pattern: Binaural beats in the theta pattern are set at a frequency of between <u>4</u> Hz and <u>8</u> Hz—which is associated with sleep in the rapid eye movement or *REM phase.*

Alpha pattern: Binaural beats in the alpha pattern are set at a frequency of between 8 Hz and 13 Hz—which may encourage *wakeful relaxation* that is ideal for learning and studying.

Beta pattern: Binaural beats in the beta pattern are set at a frequency of between 14 Hz and 100 Hz—which may help promote *concentration and alertness*. However, this frequency can also increase *anxiety* at the higher end of the frequency range (why the alpha pattern is better for learning and studying).

For the purposes of improving your sleep, we will focus on the **delta** and **theta**.

How do you use them? It's simple. Binaural beats work by either sending a different level of sound frequency to each ear through headphones or playing one level right after the other. So the trick is to listen to them while you are completing your daily sleep-aid routine (with the sleeping methods you've learned so far).

You can buy or download some binaural beats for free online—or simply listen to them on YouTube where you can also create a playlist with one wave playing after each other.

<u>Examples:</u>
–**Theta waves:** www.youtube.com/watch?v=CreU9g302yU
–**Delta waves:** www.youtube.com/watch?v=lzBk98Gb0JU

Next, lie down on your bed after you are finished doing anything else for the night and experiment listening to the waves to "tame" your brain and all your senses.

Unless you don't have to get up early in the morning—we would advise you to listen without headphones during the night before because if you fall asleep with headphones on, you may not hear your alarm clock the next day.

Exercise: Calm Down Calamity

For today, practice combining everything that we've discussed.

- Start with the breathing exercise where you lift your hands up (open your lungs) and inhale slowly, then lower your hands slowly (relax the lungs) and exhale slowly as well. Complete <u>10</u> breathing cycles.

- Then do the child yoga pose for <u>five</u> minutes. Make sure the room is silent and that you are alone and focused.

- Finally, play some binaural beats (put the playlist on autoplay if you are using YouTube directly). Make sure you are done with all of your activities for the night and lie down while you play the waves.

Goodnight. We'll see you tomorrow!

DAY 6:

Sleep Behavioral Modification

Daily Structural Changes

One common denominator among people who suffer from chronic insomnia can be attributed to their nocturnal tendencies such as working too late, watching TV all night, or staying out until the next day. All of these activities can really inhibit your natural ability to fall asleep when you need to.

Dr. Paul Saskin, a behavioral sleep medicine expert in Missouri, believes that it is paramount to have a solid clinical schedule, thus the need to condition yourself to the different periods of the day that are changing right in front of your eyes.

Now if your biological clock is so messed up from staying up too late so many times, there are ways to remedy this. *It's simple.*

Just take note that there are <u>four main periods</u> of the day which correspond to certain behaviors and that for the <u>last period</u> of the day—there's a **red line** that shouldn't be crossed. *And what is that red line?* Well, it is the timeline you shouldn't cross so that you don't disrupt your biological clock even more.

How does it work? First, let's go through the different periods of the day and *what they should mean to you* in terms of the behavior you should adopt from now on:

First period, morning: Spanning from 6 a.m. to 12 noon. This is when you should opt to work out, perform your morning ritual, and get ready for the rest of your day. Overall, this is the period when you should be the most alert and active, but most importantly, knock out your most important tasks for the day or at work, *etc.*

Second period, afternoon: Spanning from 12 noon to 6 p.m. This is when the rest of your energy levels should be allocated to your remaining daily activities like completing your work tasks and devoting to stuff outside of work.

Third period, evening: Spanning from 6 p.m. to 9 p.m. This is when you could possibly revisit what you weren't able to finish during the day, for instance, replying back to a few <u>old</u> emails or completing an <u>old</u> report, *etc.* Note the emphasis on the word "old" here— meaning only brushing up what you did today and not start anything new, because at this point you should start winding down for bed by following the previous days' recommendations like eating the right meal, taking a warm bath perhaps, having a cup of tea, and doing whatever to relax your mind before calling it a night.

Fourth period, late night: Starting at 10 p.m. There should be near silence (unless of course you're using binaural beats to help you sleep) where no other activities are allowed by this time, and you should have already gone to bed.

Early Bird Conversion

If you ask most successful and productive individuals, you'll often hear how they start off their days really early before anybody else, thus you hardly ever hear them having insomnia.

Obviously, not everyone is an early bird, but that doesn't mean you can't condition yourself to be one if you choose to. It will take some work, but follow these guidelines to reset your inner "creature of (bad) habits":

1. Create a *series of small banners* as reminders that will help you become consciously self-aware to the <u>four periods</u> of the day.

2. On the banners, write "**Morning 6 a.m. – 12 noon:** *Very active*" (Keeping in mind any important activity should fall within this time frame), "**Afternoon 12 noon – 6 p.m.:** *Still very active*" (Again, with the rest of your energy you should carry on with your important activities.), "**Evening 6 p.m. – 9 p.m.:** *Light activities*" (Slow down and start prep for sleep. You can complete unfinished tasks that are urgent, but this time frame is mostly reserved for eating your evening meal, and getting ready for bed.), and "**Late night 10 p.m.:** *Total silence*" (You should be sleeping until the alarm goes off the next day).

3. Make sure to write the banners in **bold and big letters**. Mentally ingrain them into your mind by placing these banners in strategic places (the fridge, the

wall in front of your desk, the door at work, *etc.*). Be sure to carry over what each period of the day represents *into* your performance for the next two days.

4. After two days, you can take this further by listing out the activities you must do on each banner or by occasionally checking the time on your watch, phone or clock. Whenever you glance at the time, you should adopt the behavior that *corresponds* to that particular time frame. For example, if your watch says it's **4 p.m.,** then you know that you should keep on working as hard as you have all day. Then again, if you check the time and it's **8:30 p.m.,** this means that you should now put on your pajamas, prepare your cup of tea, and grab a book to read in bed while you sip on your sleep-aid tea or warm milk.

It goes without saying that once you convert over to being an early bird—going to bed early will come naturally as a byproduct.

Exercise: Set Each Period's Performance Level

For Day 6, practice on reprogramming your performance mode so you'll know when to be *active* and when to *rest*— by placing meanings on <u>each period</u> of the day (for example, from 6 a.m. to 12 noon you should be *very active*, etc.).

Then, take it up a notch by listing your need-to-do activities or using your watch during the day for the same purpose, and every time you move into a new period of the day, you should adjust your behavior to that period.

DAY 7:

Sleep Pattern Establishment

Relaxation Therapy

We saved the best part of this seven-day sleep regimen for the last day—and that is learning to *relax*. Relaxing sounds simple on the surface but can be somewhat challenging in itself when you are very stressed and anxious to move on with the rest of your day.

But there is one simple thing you can always count on. *What is it?* Wait for it, wait for it...your bathtub. *That's right!* Taking a bath is a superior way to relax than just sitting down on the couch because the warmth and the water make the process serendipitous. *Why?*

- Warm water makes you more comfortable, thus helping you to relax.

- Normally after finishing a nice warm bath, you should feel a bit dizzy (but in a beneficial way). The dizziness is due to the fact that you've left the bathtub and entered a cooler room, which according to Dr. Joyce Walsleben, associate professor at the New York University Department of Medicine, signals your body that it's time to rest by slowing down your essential metabolic functions such as heart rate, breathing, and digestion.

To get the maximum effect from your bath, use bubbles or essential oils (involving the scents from Day 3: lavender, chamomile, bergamot, jasmine, or rose) and stay in the tub 20 to 30 minutes and, of course, make sure the water stays warm the whole time.

For more enjoyment and enhancing the experience you should:

1. Set a timer for 20-30 minutes.

2. Fold up a towel and place it under your neck like a pillow.

3. Encourage calmness and relaxation by stretching your legs forward and stretching your arms to the side.

4. Keep your eyes closed and slowly count to 30 to relax. Breathe slowly throughout the whole time, forcing yourself not to think about anything. Just think of a blank image and relax.

5. Remain in that state until your time is up.

You will notice that you'll feel a bit drowsy after being in the tub, which is a good sign. You should then proceed with the rest of your sleep preparation that we've given you (sleep-aid beverages, sleepwear, temperature in your room, *etc.*).

Now that we've walked you through the seven days—it's time to activate this entire plan. Coming next are some remaining **sleep assessment exercises** for you.

Sleep Assessment Exercise 1: Break Habits

Work on changing up your old habitual behaviors.

Prepare <u>three</u> small banners: one for your kitchen, one for your bedroom, and one for your workplace. On these banners fill in the activities that correspond to:

–**Morning from** 6 a.m. to 12 noon.

–**Afternoon from** 12 noon to 6 p.m.

–**Evening from** 6 p.m. to 9 p.m.

–**Late night** beginning at 10 p.m.

When the banners are done, start memorizing what you've classified as **morning activities** and the ones you've classified as **night activities**, then condition yourself to follow through with them to better situate yourself when it comes to getting the sleep you need.

Sleep Assessment Exercise 2: Rest Body

Before you get on to your nightly ritual, prepare a warm bath. Pour the bubbles into the water as it fills the tub. When you turn off the water, you may also consider adding three drops of the essential oil of your choice.

- Set the timer for 20-30 minutes, and then get in the bathtub.

- Put a folded towel behind your neck for comfort.

- Let yourself go and relax breathing slowly (if necessary, count to 30).

Afterward, evaluate your state:

–How would you grade your drowsiness after your bath? Very drowsy, mildly drowsy, or only a little drowsy?

–How do you feel after the bath? Are you motivated to do anything or ready to crash?

Sleep Assessment Exercise 3: Follow Routine

Set up a "go-to-sleep" routine every day by 8:30 p.m.

1. Begin by preparing your cup of sleep-aid beverage, with chamomile tea or warm milk as options.

2. Adjust the temperature in the room. Just like the porridge in the story of "Goldilocks and the Three

Bears," you don't want it to be too hot or too cold. You want it to be *just right*!

3. Get out of your clothes and put on your pajamas.

4. Give your pillow a few sprays of pillow mist.

5. Sip your beverage while doing your favorite relaxing pastimes.

6. Finally, turn off the lights and put on your night light.

From now on, this should be your routine for the final minutes of every day.

Sleep Assessment Exercise 4: Automate Activities

Now we're going to see if you've been paying attention by quizzing you about the four periods of the day. Answer these questions to see if you've prepared yourself enough these past few days in order to reprogram your performance mode:

–If you look at your watch and it's **11 a.m.**—how should you behave?

–If you consult your watch, once again, during the day and you see that it is **3 p.m.**—how should you behave?

–If you check the time and see that it's **8 p.m.**—*what activities* best suit this period of the day, and *why?*

Sleep Assessment Exercise 5: Relieve Muscles

Practice the child yoga pose by folding your lower legs under you, rolling your torso forward, and bringing your forehead to rest on the bed.

Next, lower your chest as close to your knees as you comfortably can and extend your arms in front of you.

Make sure you hold the pose and breathe. (You should actually hold the pose close to <u>five</u> minutes, again by breathing slowly while stretching the muscles on your back.)

Final Experimentation: Week Schedule Ahead

After you've learned these strategies and methods during the week, you will have to *integrate* them into your **everyday routine** from now on. We've set up a little sleep-aid schedule (with everything you've learned this week simplified) for your **second week**:

<u>DAY 1</u>:

In the morning, (from **6 a.m.** to **12 noon**), conduct your normal flow of activities, and do the same thing during the afternoon time period (from **12 noon** to **6 p.m.**) with the same intensity of activities.

Remember to *check the time* every now and then so that you remember to adopt the right behavior for the <u>time period</u>

you're in. In the evening (from **6 p.m.** to **8 p.m.**), eat dinner *(don't forget to avoid foods that are too sugary or fatty)* and introduce jasmine rice into your meal. Drink a glass of tart cherry juice after dinner and have a banana for dessert. By **8:30 p.m.**, proceed with the "go-to-sleep" routine, by enjoying a cup of chamomile tea.

Next:

1. Adjust the temperature in your bedroom.

2. Take a quick shower.

3. Put on your sleepwear.

4. Spray your pillow mist a few times on your pillow and enjoy the scent by breathing deeply a few times.

5. After you are finished drinking your tea and pastimes, turn off the lights and let yourself fall asleep.

DAY 2:

Follow the same routine regarding the different <u>time periods</u> throughout the day. But change up the meal a bit; perhaps introduce turkey into your dinner. Then by **8:30 p.m.**, move on to the "go-to-sleep" routine, with a cup of warm milk ready to sip.

Next:

1. Adjust the temperature in your bedroom.

2. Take a quick shower.

3. Put on your sleepwear.

4. Spray your pillow mist a few times on your pillow and enjoy the scent by breathing deeply a few times.

5. After you are finished drinking your milk and pastimes, turn off the lights and let yourself fall asleep.

DAY 3:

Follow the same routine regarding the different <u>time periods</u> throughout the day. At dinnertime, don't forget to avoid foods that are too rich in fat or sugar. And be sure to stay away from caffeine or alcohol. Have a glass of tart cherry juice with your evening meal or after dinner.

When you are finished eating and drinking, proceed with the "go-to-sleep" routine, but this time start with a <u>20</u> to <u>30</u> minute relaxing bath *instead* of a shower. Then prepare a cup of tea.

Next:

1. Adjust the temperature in your bedroom.

2. Put on your sleepwear.

3. Spray your pillow mist a few times on your pillow and enjoy the scent by breathing deeply a few times.

4. After you are finished drinking your tea and pastimes, turn off the lights and let yourself fall asleep.

DAY 4:

Follow the same routine regarding the different <u>time periods</u> throughout the day. At dinnertime, have jasmine rice as a part of the meal. Drink a glass of tart cherry juice after dinner and enjoy a banana for dessert.

By **8:30 p.m.**, proceed with what is the most interesting part of your day and the "go-to-sleep" routine:

1. Prepare your cup of tea and cover it to keep it warm.

2. Tidy up your bedroom a little in order to let air flow in for the next minutes (follow the guidelines we gave

for decluttering for better sleep at night). This should take only <u>10 minutes</u> or less.

3. By now, you should have one of the recommended sleep-aid plants to help you sleep better (like snake plant or aloe vera).

4. Adjust the temperature in your room.

5. Take a quick shower.

6. Put on your sleepwear.

7. Spray your pillow mist a few times on your pillow and enjoy the scent by breathing deeply a few times.

8. After you are finished drinking your tea and pastimes, turn off the lights and let yourself fall asleep.

DAY 5:

Follow the same routine regarding the different <u>time periods</u> throughout the day. At dinnertime, include a side dish of jasmine rice. Drink a glass of tart cherry juice after dinner and eat a banana for dessert.

By **8:30 p.m.**, proceed with the "go-to-sleep" routine:

1. Adjust the temperature in your room.

2. Take a quick shower.

3. Put on your sleepwear.

4. Spray your pillow mist a few times on your pillow and enjoy the scent by breathing deeply a few times.

5. Do the first yoga pose (the *wide-angle seated pose*). The session should last for <u>five minutes</u>.

6. Listen to your binaural beats playlist.

7. Turn off the lights and go to sleep.

DAY 6:

Follow the same routine regarding the different <u>time periods</u> throughout the day. Have turkey with your dinner tonight. Then by **8:30 p.m.**, move on to the "go-to-sleep" routine, with a cup of warm milk.

Next:

1. Take a warm bath for 20 to 30 minutes.

2. Adjust the temperature in your room.

3. Put on your pajamas.

4. Spray your pillow mist a few times on your pillow and enjoy the scent by breathing deeply a few times.

5. After you are done drinking your milk, turn off all the lights and let yourself fall asleep.

DAY 7:

One last time, follow the same routine regarding the different time periods throughout the day. At dinnertime, eat something light and don't forget to avoid foods that are too rich in fat or sugar. And be sure to stay away from caffeine or alcohol. Have a glass of tart cherry juice with your meal.

By 8:30 p.m., proceed with the "go-to-sleep" routine:

1. Adjust the temperature in your room.

2. Prepare a bowl of fortified cereal.

3. Put your nightwear on.

4. Eat your cereal as a sleep-aid snack along with a small glass of water.

5. Spray your pillow mist a few times on your pillow and enjoy the scent by breathing deeply a few times.

6. Do the second yoga pose (the *locust pose*). The session should last around <u>five minutes</u>.

7. Once you are done with yoga, listen to your binaural beats playlist.

8. Then, turn off all the lights and let yourself fall asleep.

Regardless of how repetitive all this might seem—ideally, it should become your routine during the evening if you want to regain healthy sleeping reflexes and hopefully sleep much better, and for longer hours.

Challenge Complete:

Awaken Refreshed

For people who suffer from anxiety and stress *(who doesn't?)* and sometimes those who work late and need coffee to stay productive, getting a good night's sleep is almost unheard of. In a way, sleeping is like a rare gem that they can no longer get their hands on.

Well, the remedy to this is quite simple. Just throw away everything toxic (even coffee) and opt for food that promotes better sleep, such as bananas, fortified cereals, and even cherries. And to make it even more interesting, you can also enhance your sleeping with aromatherapy scents like rose, lavender, chamomile, and many others.

There's also the practical application side of sleeping that you will have to experiment and explore by using binaural beats to naturally ease yourself into a deep sleep-like state with delta and theta waves, as well as carefully selecting and displaying your sleepwear so that the idea of getting to sleep becomes more inviting and possible.

You should also enjoy the experience by using it as an opportunity and excuse to take warm baths as much as possible for the natural drowsy sensation that it gives you, which will help you "surrender to the night."

Now is your time to reclaim your natural sleeping reflexes. Follow everything you have learned within these seven days, and we'll see you in dreamland! Good night!

<u>Your Feedback:</u>

Was Your Challenge Accomplished?

Congratulations on completing all your challenges! You should be proud of yourself for making it this far. For that, give yourself a big pat on the back! :)

Now, we have a huge favor that we would like to ask you. We want to know: have you accomplished the goal you established when you began this trial?

No two people are the same, so results will always vary.

If you have seen the results you wanted, give yourself another pat on the back, and please kindly share your testimonial wherever you purchased this book. If you let us know about it, we have a small free gift to offer you as a token of our appreciation.

However, if you aren't satisfied in any way, we urge you to please contact us directly to let us know what could have been different to help you achieve better results. We want to know if there is any way we can further help you.

Plus we are very easy to get a hold of online!

Official Website:

http://www.ChallengeSelf.com

Social Media:

https://www.facebook.com/ChallengeSelf

https://twitter.com/MyChallengeSelf

https://plus.google.com/+Challengeself

"YOU" are our main priority, and we're all here for you!

Take care! And always challenge yourself!